Concurrent substance use and mental health disorders
An information guide

W.J. Wayne Skinner, MSW, RSW; Caroline P. O'Grady, RN, MN, PhD
Christina Bartha, MSW, CSW; Carol Parker, MSW, CSW

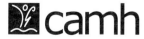

Centre for Addiction and Mental Health
Centre de toxicomanie et de santé mentale
A Pan American Health Organization /
World Health Organization Collaborating Centre

Library and Archives Canada Cataloguing in Publication

Concurrent substance use and mental health disorders : an information guide / W.J. Wayne Skinner ... [et al.].

Issued also in electronic formats.

1. Dual diagnosis. 2. Mentally ill--Alcohol use. 3. Mentally ill--Drug use. 4. Substance abuse. 5. Mental illness. I. Skinner, W. J. Wayne, 1949- II. Centre for Addiction and Mental Health

RC564.68.C65 2011   616.86   C2011-901557-9

ISBN: 978-1-77052-603-7 (PRINT)
ISBN: 978-1-77052-604-4 (PDF)
ISBN: 978-1-77052-605-1 (HTML)
ISBN: 978-1-77052-606-8 (ePUB)

Printed in Canada
Copyright © 2004, 2010 Centre for Addiction and Mental Health

No part of this work may be reproduced or transmitted in any form or by any means electronic or mechanical, including photocopying and recording, or by any information storage and retrieval system without written permission from the publisher—except for a brief quotation (not to exceed 200 words) in a review or professional work.

This publication may be available in other formats. For information about alternate formats or other CAMH publications, or to place an order, please contact Sales and Distribution:
Toll-free: 1 800 661-1111
Toronto: 416 595-6059
E-mail: publications@camh.net
Online store: http://store.camh.net

Website: www.camh.net

Disponible en français sous le titre : Les troubles concomitants de toxicomanie et de santé mentale.

This guide was produced by the following:
Development: Caroline Hebblethwaite, CAMH
Editorial: Nick Gamble, CAMH; Kelly Coleman
Graphic design: Nancy Leung, CAMH
Print production: Christine Harris, CAMH

3973i / 06-2011 / PM039

Contents

Authorship v

Acknowledgment vi

Introduction vi

1 What are concurrent disorders? 1
   How common are concurrent disorders?
   When do concurrent disorders begin?

2 What are the symptoms of concurrent disorders? 5
   How severe are the problems?
   How does each problem affect the other one?

3 What causes concurrent disorders? 9

4 How are concurrent disorders treated? 10
   Where do people get treatment?
   What is integrated treatment?
   Treatment goals
   Types of treatment
   Special treatment situations

5 Recovery and relapse prevention 28
   What does it mean to be "in recovery"?
   Preventing relapse and promoting wellness

6 How concurrent disorders affect families 32
   What happens when someone you love has concurrent disorders?
   Getting treatment for your family member
   Care for families
   Being ready for a relapse or crisis
   Tips for helping your family member

7   Explaining concurrent disorders to children   40
How much should I tell the children?
What to tell children
Outside the home
During illness
During recovery

Reference   45

Resources   46

Authorship

The Client and Family Information Guide series originated in the Social Work Department of the Clarke Institute of Psychiatry, one of the four organizations that merged in 1998 to form the Centre for Addiction and Mental Health (CAMH). Since then, these guides have become an important part of the CAMH publishing program.

Concurrent disorders is a relatively new field. To learn about it, we have drawn on the wisdom of people from a wide variety of mental health and substance use backgrounds. We thank the author teams who produced the other guides in this series:

Christina Bartha
Pamela Blake
Dale Butterill
David Clodman
April Collins
Robert Cooke
Donna Czuchta
Dave Denberg
Martin Katzman
Kate Kitchen
Stephanie Kruger

Alice Kusznir
Roger McIntyre
Sagar Parikh
Carol Parker
Jane Paterson
Neil Rector
Margaret Richter
Kathryn Ryan
Mary Seeman
Cathy Thomson
Claudia Tindall

Collaboration with CAMH Publication Services has been essential in creating this guide. Caroline Hebblethwaite and Anita Dubey deserve special recognition for their expertise and skill in producing this guide.

Acknowledgment

The authors would like to pay special tribute to clients at CAMH and their families who, through their openness, have taught us so much.

Introduction

This guide is for people with concurrent disorders and for their families. It is also for anyone who wants basic information about concurrent disorders, their treatment and their management. This guide should not replace treatment from a health professional.

The term "concurrent disorders" covers many combinations of problems. This guide talks about issues that are common to most concurrent disorders. Other guides in the series offer more details about specific mental health problems (see page 51 for a list of titles).

1 What are concurrent disorders?

A person with a mental health problem has a higher risk of having a substance use problem, just as a person with a substance use problem has an increased chance of having a mental health problem. People who have combined, or concurrent, substance use and mental health problems are said to have *concurrent disorders*.

Concurrent disorders can include combinations such as:

- an anxiety disorder and a drinking problem
- schizophrenia and addiction to cannabis
- borderline personality disorder and heroin addiction
- depression and addiction to sleeping pills.

(Addiction can be defined as the presence of the 4 Cs: Craving, loss of Control of the amount or frequency of use, Compulsion to use, and use despite negative Consequences.)

Many other concurrent disorders are possible, because there are many types of mental health and substance use problems.

A NOTE ABOUT LANGUAGE

In this information guide, we use the phrases "substance use problem" or "mental health problem" to describe the broad range of situations, from mild to severe, that a person with concurrent disorders may experience. We use the phrases "substance use disorder" or "mental health disorder" only where the text refers to a specific diagnosis.

Concurrent disorders are also sometimes called:

- dual disorders
- dual diagnosis
- co-occurring substance use and mental health problems.

In Ontario, the term *dual diagnosis* is used when a person has an intellectual disability and a mental health problem.

How common are concurrent disorders?

A large American study by Reiger and colleagues (1990) found the following rates:

- 30 per cent of people diagnosed with a mental health disorder will also have a substance use disorder at some time in their lives. This is close to twice the rate found in people who do not have a lifetime history of a mental health disorder.
- 37 per cent of people diagnosed with an alcohol disorder will have a mental health disorder at some point in their lives. This is close to twice the rate found in people who do not have a lifetime history of a substance use disorder.

- 53 per cent of people diagnosed with a substance use disorder (other than alcohol) will also have a mental health disorder at some point in their lives. This is close to four times the rate found in people who do not have a lifetime history of a substance use disorder.

The most common combinations are:

- substance use disorders + anxiety disorders
- substance use disorders + mood disorders.

Anxiety disorders
- In general, 10 to 25 per cent of all people will have an anxiety disorder in their lifetime.
- Among people who have had an anxiety disorder in their lifetime, 24 per cent will have a substance use disorder in their lifetime.

Major depression
- In general, 15 to 20 per cent of all people will have major depression in their lifetime.
- Among people who have had major depression in their lifetime, 27 per cent will have a substance use disorder in their lifetime.

Bipolar disorder
- In general, one to two per cent of all people will have bipolar disorder in their lifetime.
- Among people who have had bipolar disorder in their lifetime, 56 per cent will have a substance use disorder in their lifetime.

Schizophrenia
- In general, one per cent of all people will have schizophrenia in their lifetime.
- Among people who have had schizophrenia in their lifetime, 47 per cent will have a substance use disorder in their lifetime.

When do concurrent disorders begin?

Mental health and substance use problems can begin at any time: from childhood to old age. When problems begin early and are severe, recovery will probably take longer, and the person will need to work harder and have more support. On the other hand, if the problem is caught and treated early, the person has a better chance of a quicker and fuller recovery.

People often ask, "Which came first: the mental health problem or the substance use problem?" This is a hard question to answer. Often it is more useful to think of them as independent problems that interact with each other.

2 What are the symptoms of concurrent disorders?

Concurrent disorders is a term for any combination of mental health and substance use problems. There is no one symptom or group of symptoms that is common to all combinations.

The combinations of concurrent disorders can be divided into five main groups:

- substance use + mood and anxiety disorders, such as depression or panic disorder
- substance use + severe and persistent mental health disorders, such as schizophrenia or bipolar disorder
- substance use + personality disorders, such as borderline personality disorder, or problems related to anger, impulsivity or aggression
- substance use + eating disorders, such as anorexia nervosa or bulimia
- other substance use + mental health disorders, such as gambling and sexual disorders.

To understand and treat a particular combination, we need to look at the specific problems to see:

- how severe the problems are
- how the problems affect each other.

How severe are the problems?

Some people with concurrent disorders have very severe problems with both their mental health and their substance use. This makes it hard for them to function day-to-day. While other people may have milder mental health and substance use problems, the impact on their lives can still be difficult.

People with concurrent disorders are likely to receive treatment in one of the following settings:

- primary health care; for example, family doctors
- mental health agencies
- substance use agencies
- specialized concurrent disorders treatment programs.

The treatment setting often depends on how severe a person's problems are.

What are the symptoms of concurrent disorders?

More severe substance use problems; mild to moderate mental health problems **TREATMENT:** mainly in the substance use system	Severe substance use and mental health problems **TREATMENT:** ideally with specialized care for concurrent disorders
Milder substance use and mental health problems **TREATMENT:** in the community with a family doctor	More severe mental health problems; mild to moderate substance use problems **TREATMENT:** mainly in the mental health system

Substance Use Problems (Low severity → High severity)

Mental Health Problems (Low severity → High severity)

How does each problem affect the other one?

Mental health problems and substance use problems can affect each other in several ways:

- Substance use can make mental health problems worse.
- Substance use can mimic or hide the symptoms of mental health problems.

- Sometimes people turn to substance use to "relieve" or forget about the symptoms of mental health problems.
- Some substances can make mental health medications less effective.
- Using substances can make people forget to take their medications. If this happens, the mental health problems may come back ("relapse") or get worse.
- When a person relapses with one problem, it can trigger the symptoms of the other problem.

A person with concurrent disorders will often have more serious medical, social and emotional problems than if he or she had only one condition. Treatment may take longer and be more challenging.

3 What causes concurrent disorders?

There is no simple cause of concurrent disorders. Each person's situation is different. Here are some reasons why a person might develop both a mental health and a substance use problem:

- Some people who have a mental health problem may use substances to feel better. While substance use is very risky in such cases, it can help people forget their problems or relieve symptoms, at least in the short term. People sometimes talk about using substances for "self-medication."
- Some effects of substance use can mimic symptoms of a mental health problem, such as depression, anxiety, impulsivity or hallucinations. This is sometimes described as substance-induced mental health problems.
- Substance use can cause harmful changes in people's lives and relationships. For example, substance use problems may cause a person to lose his or her job. Mental health problems may result from these indirect effects of substance use.
- For some people, a common factor may lead to both mental health and substance use problems. This factor may be biological. It may also be an event, such as emotional or physical trauma.

For a person whose mental health is fragile, even moderate amounts of substance use may create problems.

4 How are concurrent disorders treated?

People who have concurrent disorders often have to go to one service for mental health treatment and another place for addiction treatment. Sometimes the services are not connected at all.

However, concurrent substance use and mental health problems are often related, and they affect each other. So clients have the best success when both problems are addressed at the same time, in a co-ordinated way. The treatment approach usually depends on the type and severity of the person's problems. A person might receive psychosocial treatments (individual or group therapy) or biological treatments (medications), or often both.

Although the overall treatment plan should consider both mental health and substance use problems, it is sometimes best to treat one problem first. For example, most people who have concurrent mood and alcohol disorders are likely to recover better if the alcohol disorder is treated first.

As another example, a person who is being treated for concurrent problems may have an episode in which the mental health problem gets worse. Treatment might at that point focus on the mental health problem, rather than on the substance use.

Where do people get treatment?

Most people with concurrent disorders have mild to moderate problems that can be treated in the community, through their family doctor, for example. People with severe problems may need specialized care for concurrent disorders.

What is integrated treatment?

Clients with severe concurrent mental health and substance use problems may need *integrated treatment*. Integrated treatment is a way of making sure that treatment is smooth, co-ordinated and comprehensive for the client. It ensures that the client receives help not only with the concurrent disorders, but also in other life areas, such as housing and employment. Ongoing support in these life areas helps clients to:

- maintain treatment successes
- prevent relapses
- ensure their basic life needs are being met.

Integrated treatment works best if the client has a stable, trusting, long-term relationship with one *case facilitator*. This person is a health care professional, such as a case manager or therapist. Even though one person is responsible for overseeing the client's treatment, the client may work with a team of professionals, such as psychiatrists, social workers and addiction therapists.

If all the treatment services are not in one location, two or more programs may work together to co-ordinate treatment. For example, a therapist in an addiction program might ask new clients questions to see if they also have mental health problems. If the clients do, the addiction program could either:

- treat the mental health problems, or
- refer clients to a mental health agency, and work with that agency. Therapists at both agencies would keep in touch about the clients' progress.

Treatment goals

In the past, addiction and mental health treatment services have each had different ways of treating problems. They have also had different ways of thinking about problems. Clients who received treatment from both systems may have been confused by the differences. For example:

- Many addiction services agree that *reducing* substance use is a realistic goal for clients at the beginning of treatment. This is called *harm reduction*. As the client moves through treatment, the long-term goal may be *abstinence*: to stop the use of the substance completely. However, some mental health programs ask clients to completely stop using alcohol or other drugs before they can get treatment.
- Many mental health problems benefit from treatment with medications. However, some substance use programs may try to help the client stop taking all drugs, including those used to treat mental health problems.

Fortunately, staff in many mental health and substance use programs now work more closely together. As a result, clients may see fewer differences like the ones described above.

The ultimate goal of treatment is for clients to:

- decide what a healthy future means for them
- find ways to live a healthy life.

The treatment plan needs to be customized—this means it will address each client's particular needs. Both the substance use and the mental health problems will be addressed with the most appropriate approaches from each field.

Types of treatment

Treatment for concurrent disorders includes psychosocial treatments and medication. Clients may receive one or the other, or both.

PSYCHOSOCIAL TREATMENTS

Psychosocial treatments are an important part of treatment for concurrent disorders. They include:

- psychoeducation
- psychotherapy (counselling, individual and group therapy)
- family therapy
- peer support.

Psychoeducation
Psychoeducation is education about mental health and substance use issues. People who know about their problems are more able to make informed choices. Knowledge can help clients and their families:

- deal with their problems
- make plans to prevent problems
- build a plan to support recovery.

While all people should receive psychoeducation when they begin treatment for concurrent disorders, as they move through recovery they may benefit more from psychoeducation. For people who have milder problems, psychoeducation alone may be the only treatment they need.

Psychoeducation sessions include discussions about:

- what causes substance use and mental health problems
- how the problems might be treated
- how to self-manage the problems (if possible)
- how to prevent future episodes.

Psychotherapy

Psychotherapy is sometimes called "talk therapy." It helps people deal with their problems by looking at how they:

- think
- act
- interact with others.

There are many different types of psychotherapy. Some types are better for certain problems. Psychotherapy can be either short-term or long-term.

Short-term therapy has a specific focus and structure. The therapist is active and directs the process. This type of treatment is usually no longer than 10 to 20 sessions.

In *long-term therapy*, the therapist is generally less active, and the process is less structured. The treatment usually lasts at least one year. The aim is to help the client work through deep psychological issues.

Successful therapy depends on a supportive, comfortable relationship with a trusted therapist. The therapist can be a:

- doctor
- social worker
- psychologist
- other professional.

Therapists are trained in different types of psychotherapy. They may work in hospitals, clinics or private practice.

COGNITIVE-BEHAVIOURAL THERAPY

Cognitive-behavioural therapy (CBT) is a type of short-term psychotherapy. CBT works well for a broad range of concurrent disorders.

In CBT, people learn to look at how their beliefs or thoughts affect the way they look at themselves and the world. Some deeply held thoughts have a strong influence on our mood and behaviour. For instance, if we are depressed and drinking too much and think no treatment will help, then we might not seek treatment. CBT helps people identify and change such thoughts and learn new strategies to get along better in everyday life.

DIALECTICAL BEHAVIOURAL THERAPY

Dialectical behavioural therapy (DBT) is a type of cognitive-behavioural therapy. It is used to treat a range of behaviour problems. DBT draws on Western cognitive behaviour techniques and Eastern Zen philosophies. It teaches clients how to:

- become more aware of their thoughts and actions
- tolerate distress
- manage their emotions
- improve their relationships with other people.

INSIGHT-ORIENTED OR PSYCHODYNAMIC PSYCHOTHERAPIES
Insight-oriented or psychodynamic psychotherapies tend to be longer-term and less structured. These therapies reduce distress by helping people understand what makes them act the way they do.

INTERPERSONAL THERAPY
Interpersonal therapies help clients get better at communicating and interacting with others. These therapies help people:

- look at how they interact with others
- identify issues and problems in relationships
- explore ways to make changes.

Interpersonal group therapy focuses on the interactions among group members.

GROUP THERAPY
Group therapy can help people who have concurrent disorders. Group therapy can include treatments such as:

- cognitive-behavioural therapy
- interpersonal therapy
- psychoeducation.

A group setting can be a comfortable place to discuss issues such as family relationships, medication side-effects and relapses.

Family therapy
Families may also be involved in the person's treatment. Support from family members can help the person who has concurrent disorders. Family members may also enter therapy themselves. Therapy for families can offer a range of help. For example:

- Families can learn about substance use and mental health problems.
- Family members can enter care as clients themselves.

Family therapy can:

- teach families about concurrent disorders
- offer advice and support to family members.

Usually therapists work with one family at a time. Sometimes family therapy is offered in a group setting with other families in similar situations. Group members can share feelings and experiences with other families who understand and support them.

Peer support groups

Peer support groups can be an important part of treatment. A peer support group is a group of people who all have concurrent disorders. These people can accept and understand one another, and can share their struggles in a safe, supportive environment. Group members usually develop a strong bond among themselves. People who have recently been diagnosed with concurrent disorders can benefit from the experiences of others.

There are peer support groups for clients and for families. Groups for clients include Double Trouble groups and Dual Recovery Anonymous. The Family Association for Mental Health Everywhere (FAME) has groups for families. See page 47 for further information. Although these groups are often called *self*-help, peer support actually offers a type of help called *mutual aid*.

BIOLOGICAL TREATMENTS

Medications used to treat mental health problems

The information in the following section is summarized from a series of pamphlets, entitled *Understanding Psychiatric Medications*, available from the Centre for Addiction and Mental Health. The pamphlets are designed to help people better understand and make choices about psychiatric drugs. They discuss what the drugs are used for, the different types and names of drugs, their effects and their place in the treatment of mental health problems. Online versions are available at www.camh.net.

ANTIDEPRESSANT MEDICATIONS
Antidepressant medications are used to treat depression. Some are also helpful for anxiety disorders. There are several classes of antidepressants; within each class there are many individual medications. While all antidepressants work well overall, no drug or type of drug works equally well for everyone who takes it. Some people may be advised to try another type of antidepressant or to use a combination of antidepressants to seek relief from their distress.

The different types of antidepressants are listed below in the order in which they are most commonly prescribed.

Selective serotonin reuptake inhibitors (SSRIS)
This group of drugs includes fluoxetine (Prozac), paroxetine (Paxil), fluvoxamine (Luvox), citalopram (Celexa), escitalopram (Cipralex) and sertraline (Zoloft). SSRIS are usually the first choice for treatment of depression and anxiety problems. These medications are known to have milder side-effects than some other antidepressants. Buspirone (Buspar) is similar to SSRIS and has been found to help with anxiety but not depression.

Serotonin and norepinephrine reuptake inhibitors (SNRIS)
This class of medications includes venlafaxine (Effexor), duloxetine (Cymbalta) and desvenlafaxine (Pristiq). These drugs are used to treat depression, anxiety problems and chronic pain.

Norepinephrine and dopamine reuptake inhibitors (NDRIS)
The medication available in this class is bupropion (Wellbutrin, Zyban). When used to treat depression, it is often given for its energizing effects, in combination with other antidepressants. It is also used to treat attention-deficit/hyperactivity disorder and as a smoking cessation aid.

Noradrenergic and specific serotonergic antidepressants (NASSAS)
Mirtazapine (Remeron), the medication available in this class, is the most sedating antidepressant, making it a good choice for people who have insomnia or who are very anxious. This medication also helps to stimulate appetite.

Cyclics
This older group includes amitriptyline (Elavil), maprotiline (Ludiomil), imipramine (Tofranil), desipramine (Norpramin), nortriptyline (Novo-Nortriptyline) and clomipramine (Anafranil).

Because these drugs tend to have more side-effects than the newer drugs, they are not often a first choice for treatment. However, when other drugs do not provide relief from severe depression, these drugs may help.

Monoamine oxidase inhibitors (MAOIS)
MAOIs, such as phenelzine (Nardil) and tranylcypromine (Parnate), were the first class of antidepressants. MAOIs are effective, but they are not often used because people who take them must follow a special diet.

A newer MAOI, moclobemide (Manerix), can be used without dietary restrictions; however, it may not be as effective as other MAOIS.

ANTI-ANXIETY MEDICATIONS

Anti-anxiety medications are used to treat anxiety. *Benzodiazepines* are a family of anti-anxiety medications; some are also used for insomnia. Many types of benzodiazepines are available in Canada. All benzodiazepines work the same way; however, the intensity and duration of their effects vary.

The benzodiazepines most commonly used to treat anxiety disorders are clonazepam (Rivotril), alprazolam (Xanax) and lorazepam (Ativan). Also used are bromazepam (Lectopam), oxazepam (Serax), chlordiazepoxide (once marketed as Librium), clorazepate (Tranxene) and diazepam (Valium).

Benzodiazepines used for the treatment of insomnia include lorazepam (Ativan), nitrazepam (Mogadon), oxazepam (Serax), temazepam (Restoril), triazolam (Halcion) and flurazepam (Dalmane).

Another drug used for insomnia is zopiclone (Imovane). This drug is similar to benzodiazepines and has similar side-effects. Zopiclone may have less abuse potential than some benzodiazepines; however, people can still become addicted to this drug.

MOOD STABILIZERS

Mood stabilizers are medicines that help reduce mood swings. They also help prevent manic and depressive episodes. The oldest and most studied of the mood stabilizers is lithium. Lithium is a simple element in the same family as sodium (table salt). Many drugs that were first developed as anticonvulsants to treat epilepsy also act as mood stabilizers. These include carbamazepine (Tegretol), divalproex (Epival) and lamotrigine (Lamictal). Gabapentin (Neurontin) and topiramate (Topamax) are also anticonvulsants that may act as mood stabilizers, although they are usually only given in addition to other medications.

Some people may be prescribed more than one type of mood stabilizer to take in combination.

ANTIPSYCHOTIC MEDICATIONS
Antipsychotic medications are used to treat psychosis. Delusions and hallucinations are examples of symptoms of psychosis. Antipsychotic medications are generally divided into two categories: first generation (*typical*) and second generation (*atypical*). Both categories of drugs work equally well overall, although no drug or type of drug works equally well for everyone who takes it.

Antipsychotics are often used in combination with other medications to treat other symptoms of mental health problems or to offset side-effects.

Most people who take antipsychotics over a longer term are now prescribed the second-generation drugs.

Second-generation (atypical) antipsychotics
Medications available in this class include risperidone (Risperdal), quetiapine (Seroquel), olanzapine (Zyprexa), ziprasidone (Zeldox), paliperidone (Invega), aripiprazole (Abilify) and clozapine (Clozaril). Clozapine is exceptional in that it often works even when other medications have failed; however, because it requires monitoring of white blood cell counts, it is not the first choice for treatment.

First-generation (typical) antipsychotics
These older medications include chlorpromazine (once marketed as Largactil), flupenthixol (Fluanxol), fluphenazine (Modecate), haloperidol (Haldol), loxapine (Loxapac), perphenazine (Trilafon), pimozide (Orap), trifluoperazine (Stelazine), thiothixene (Navane) and zuclopenthixol (Clopixol).

Medications used to treat substance use problems

Medications can also help treat substance use problems. Some are used in the short term while others may be needed for longer periods.

There are three main types of medications that help with substance use:

- aversive medications
- medications that reduce cravings
- substitution medications.

AVERSIVE MEDICATIONS

People who take *aversive medications* will have unpleasant effects if they continue their substance use. An example of an aversive medication is disulfiram (Antabuse), which is used for alcohol addiction.

CRAVING REDUCTION

Some medications change the way brain chemicals respond to drugs. They may block the enjoyable effects of a drug, or reduce cravings for the drug. Examples of *medications that reduce cravings* are:

- naltrexone (ReVia) for alcohol or opioid addiction
- bupropion (Wellbutrin, Zyban) for nicotine addiction.

SUBSTITUTION MEDICATIONS

Substitution medications reduce or prevent withdrawal symptoms. They may also reduce or eliminate drug cravings. Combined with medical and social support, these medications can help people leave the lifestyle that revolves around harmful substance use. Methadone, used to treat addiction to opioid drugs such as heroin, is the most common substitution medication.

Compliance and side-effects

Medications may have troubling side-effects. Many side-effects lessen with time. If you are having serious side-effects, talk to your doctor. The doctor can change the dose or prescribe other medications to reduce or avoid side-effects. Remember, too, that substance use may interfere with the positive effects of medications.

A doctor will monitor your use of medication. In some cases, the doctor may check the amount of medication in your blood. This allows you to receive the correct dose. The doctor may also check some body organs to see how they are affected by medication.

With the proper precautions, the risk of serious complications from medications is usually lower than the risks of living with untreated substance use and/or mental health problems.

Special treatment situations

During their recovery, people may need specific interventions, such as:

- withdrawal management
- crisis management
- relapse prevention
- hospitalization.

WITHDRAWAL MANAGEMENT

People sometimes need short-term help with withdrawal from substance use. *Withdrawal management* helps them manage symptoms that happen when they stop using the substance. Withdrawal management helps prepare clients for long-term treatment. Clients also learn about substance use and treatment options.

There are three types of withdrawal management:

- In community withdrawal management, the person goes through withdrawal at home. Health care professionals help support and guide the person through this.
- A person may stay in a withdrawal management centre. This is a special facility where the person receives more intensive care and supervision.
- Medical withdrawal management may be needed if a client has severe withdrawal symptoms, such as seizures or hallucinations. A doctor and nurse supervise the withdrawal. The client may stay in hospital or visit as an outpatient. The client may receive medications to replace the drug or ease symptoms.

CRISIS MANAGEMENT

There may be times when people who have concurrent disorders are *in crisis*. For example, the person may be in danger of hurting himself or herself, or other people.

It can be very hard for family members to cope effectively with a sudden crisis. It is useful to plan some emergency strategies when the person is well. This allows everyone to be prepared if anything does happen.

Depending on the situation, a crisis may be managed at home with family, peer and professional support. Sometimes, the person may need to be hospitalized as a result of a crisis.

After the crisis has passed, the person may need a change in the treatment approach. The person may need to return to therapy if he or she has finished treatment.

RELAPSE PREVENTION

In their most severe forms, mental health and substance use problems are chronic and recurring. This means that, even after a person has received treatment, the problems may come back, or *relapse*.

Relapse is part of the recovery process. A relapse is not a reason to stop treatment. If the person is taking medications for a mental health problem, he or she needs to keep taking them.

It is important to acknowledge and discuss the relapse. Relapse can be used as a chance to learn, to review the treatment plan and to renew a plan of action.

People who have had a relapse of substance use or mental health problems may not need intensive medical care. The relapse may be handled through individual therapy or in a group setting.

HOSPITALIZATION

During a severe crisis or relapse, some people may need to be in the hospital. This may be when clients are at risk of serious consequences, due to:

- aggressive behaviour
- taking dangerous risks
- overdosing
- self-harming or suicidal behaviour
- failing to look after their own basic needs.

In such cases, the person may stay in the hospital from a few days up to a few weeks. In hospital, the person may attend group or individual therapy sessions each day. Clients should expect to leave hospital when:

- follow-up arrangements are in place
- symptoms have improved
- they are able to function safely and care for themselves at home.

Voluntary versus involuntary admissions

People are usually admitted to hospital *voluntarily*. This means that they:

- agreed to enter the hospital
- are free to leave the hospital at any time.

However, in most places, the law also allows any doctor to admit a person to hospital *involuntarily*. This means the person may not agree that he or she needs help, and does not want to be in the hospital. Involuntary admission can happen if the doctor believes there is a serious risk that:

- the person will physically harm himself or herself
- the person will physically harm someone else.

Each province, state or jurisdiction has its own process for admitting people to hospital involuntarily. For example, in Ontario, if the person doesn't have a doctor, families may ask a justice of the peace to order an examination by a physician. In the examination, the physician will decide if the person needs to be assessed in a hospital with a psychiatric facility. The physician must be able to prove that the person's illness represents a risk of harm.

Laws protect the rights of people who are admitted involuntarily. For instance, a "rights advisor" will visit. The rights advisor will ensure that the person has the chance to appeal the involuntary status before an independent board of lawyers, doctors and laypeople.

The police are sometimes needed to help to get a person to hospital. Family members may agonize over whether to involve the police. They often feel very guilty about calling the police, even if the police are needed to protect the person's life. Remember, when people threaten suicide, they are usually pleading for help. They are taken seriously. Suicidal thinking is often a temporary feeling. When a person feels suicidal, he or she needs to be kept safe.

5 Recovery and relapse prevention

Some people with concurrent disorders may feel as if they have too many problems. They may feel these problems are too much to overcome, and that life will never be good again. They may also feel unable to do all the things they did before.

These feelings are natural and understandable. Yet, treatment, support and effort can help people with concurrent disorders to live meaningful, rewarding lives.

One of the first steps toward recovery is to set appropriate goals and priorities. This often happens during treatment, but recovery can also happen without the help of professionals.

Family members are also important during recovery. It can help if you talk about your plans and concerns with family to receive their support and feedback.

What does it mean to be "in recovery"?

Each person has a different idea about what recovery means. The key goals of treatment are:

- managing mental health symptoms
- reducing or ending substance use
- reducing the risk of relapse
- improving work life and relationships.

Many people measure recovery by their success in meeting these goals. However, recovery is more than this. Recovery is a process; it depends as much on attitude as it does on following a treatment plan. The process of recovery can include:

- developing self-confidence
- feeling hopeful and optimistic about the future
- setting achievable goals
- making changes to your housing, lifestyle or employment situation.

A client in recovery is not "cured." People may still have symptoms and struggle with their problems during their recovery. A relapse of substance use or mental health problems is often part of the process.

Recovery takes time. You may expect to have at least a year of care as part of your recovery, and to be involved in different programs in different settings.

Preventing relapse and promoting wellness

The following tips may help you prevent relapse and have a healthy lifestyle.

1. **Become an expert on your condition.** Ask your treatment provider about your problems and their treatment. Many resources are available. These include:

   - books
   - videos
   - support groups
   - information on the Internet.

   The quality of information varies. Ask your treatment team to recommend good sources.

2. **Stick to your plan to manage both problems.** This includes:

   - taking medications as prescribed
   - avoiding situations or people that might trigger substance use
   - attending treatment sessions
   - taking good care of yourself.

3. **Live a healthy life.** Eat a healthy diet, sleep well and exercise. Regular exercise can positively affect mood. Try to follow a regular routine that includes activities in the evenings and on weekends. Use your faith, religion or healing practices that support your recovery.

4. **You can't get rid of stress, so find ways to cope with stress.** Many people use only one *coping strategy*, or way to deal with stress. Work with your treatment team to find strategies to handle day-to-day stress.

5. **Have a support network of family and friends.** A strong social network can be a big support. You can nurture and build this network to help protect you from situations that cause stress. Friends or family may recognize symptoms of mental health problems or situations that trigger substance use; they can assist you in seeking help if necessary.

6. **Watch for signs of mental health problems or urges to use substances, and ask for help if you need it.** You may be able to sense early signs of an episode of illness, or the urge to use substances again. Seeking help at these times may prevent a relapse. If a relapse does happen, getting help may prevent things from getting worse.

7. **Try to balance your life.** Remember to do things in moderation. Divide your time among:

    - work
    - family
    - friends
    - leisure activities.

    A balanced and satisfying life can help you cope with stress. It may reduce your risk of relapse.

8. **Remember how and why you need to stay well.** Remind yourself of the things that help you stay well and the reasons for doing so. Reminders can include things like:

    - carrying photographs of loved ones in your wallet
    - keeping a list of positive things in your life.

    It may also be helpful to carry a list of activities that support recovery, as well as emergency numbers to contact in a crisis.

6 How concurrent disorders affect families

What happens when someone you love has concurrent disorders?

When someone has any chronic problem, it affects his or her entire family. Family members must cope with extra stressors.

Many family members struggle to accept that their relative has both substance use and mental health problems. Some families may accept the mental health diagnosis, but not the substance use problem. They may think the substance use is a sign of "bad" behaviour. Other families may accept the substance use, but find it hard to accept that their relative has a mental health problem. Some families struggle to understand that concurrent disorders are a relapsing condition, and not an illness with a cure.

Family members may feel:

- guilt
- shame
- grief
- depression
- anxiety
- a sense of loss.

They need to recognize that the expectations they had for their family member may change.

However, families can play a strong role in recovery. With support and understanding from families, people with concurrent disorders are more likely to have a successful and lasting recovery.

Family members need to learn how to:

- communicate effectively
- help when needed
- know when to let go
- take care of themselves.

As the relative undergoes treatment, family members may also feel hope and optimism. They may begin to appreciate how hard it is for their relative and admire the person's courage. When the person with concurrent disorders has success in treatment, family members may also feel a sense of personal reward.

Getting treatment for your family member

It may be hard to get your relative or partner to accept help. The person may be so discouraged about the situation that he or she may not be able to see how treatment might help. People with concurrent disorders are more likely than other people to have other health care issues. But they may not have a diagnosis of concurrent disorders. So, even though you may suspect the nature of the problem, your relative might refuse to accept that he or she needs treatment for concurrent disorders.

It is best to be supportive when trying to get your relative to accept help. It is not helpful to be confrontational. One way to be supportive about getting help is to find where your relative is least resistant to the idea of changing. For example, the person may mention that drinking has a terrible effect on his or her mood. You could then start talking about drinking. You could use this discussion to start the person thinking about getting help.

When your family member is ready to seek treatment, take an active role in helping. An active role could involve, for example:

- finding treatment centres
- setting up an appointment
- coming to the appointment.

With the consent of your family member, you may also be able to give the therapist information that offers insight into the person's situation.

Care for families

When someone has a serious condition, family members naturally feel worried and stressed. They spend time comforting or helping their loved one. At the same time, they are also dealing with the usual challenges of family life. As a result:

- They may find that caring for their family member has replaced their own routines and activities.
- They may be unsure of how others may respond to the person with concurrent disorders, so they avoid having friends visit their home.
- Over time, they may lose touch with their own network of friends.

RECOGNIZE SIGNS OF STRESS

You need to recognize signs of stress in yourself. Often, people take a long time to realize how emotionally and physically drained they have become. This stress can lead to:

- sleeping badly
- feeling exhausted all the time
- feeling irritable all the time.

RECOGNIZE YOUR OWN FEELINGS

Your own feelings are important. If you accept your own feelings, you can better help the person who has the concurrent disorders. You may feel:

- sad that the person has both a substance use and a mental health problem
- angry that this has happened to your relative and seriously affects you as well
- afraid of what the future holds
- worried about how you will cope
- guilty—that somehow you caused the problem
- a deep sense of loss when your relative behaves in ways that you do not recognize
- stressed by the extra tasks you have to take on.

TAKE CARE OF YOURSELF

You need to look after your own physical and mental health. To do this, you need to:

- Find your own limits.
- Make time for yourself. Keep up your interests outside the family and apart from your relative.
- Think about people you might want to confide in. Substance use and mental health problems are hard for some people to understand.
- Be careful—confide only in people who will support you.
- Consider seeking support for yourself, even if your relative is not in treatment. Understanding your relative's problems and the impact they have on you will help you cope better. Perhaps join a self-help organization or family support program. Local community mental health clinics, substance use treatment agencies or hospitals may offer such programs.
- Acknowledge and accept that sometimes you will have negative feelings about the situation. These feelings are normal—try not to feel guilty about them.

Being ready for a relapse or crisis

Families often avoid talking to their relative about relapses or crises. They fear that talking about a crisis will bring one on, or will upset their relative. Also, everyone hopes that the last crisis was something that only happened once, and will not happen again.

However, the best way to handle a crisis, or possibly avoid one, is to know what to do before it happens. While you focus on wellness, you should also plan for a crisis or relapse. This can help both the ill person and the family to feel more secure.

When your relative or partner is well, plan what to do if problems come back. Consider the following:

- Could you both visit the doctor to discuss your relative's condition and how to deal with a possible crisis?
- Will your relative give you advance permission to contact his or her doctor?
- Do you have your relative's consent to take him or her to hospital in a crisis? If so, which hospital has your relative chosen?
- If your relative becomes ill and cannot decide on treatment, does he or she agree that you can decide?

You may want to write down the terms that you and your relative have agreed on. This can help to ensure that the terms are followed. You can also build a good relationship with a therapist and have a prearranged emergency plan to avoid a crisis.

Tips for helping your family member

1. **Learn as much as you can about the causes, signs and symptoms, and treatment of the problems your family member has.** This will help you to understand and support your family member in recovery.

    Acknowledge and accept your own feelings. Having conflicting emotions is normal. Knowing this can help you control these emotions, so you can support your relative through recovery.

2. **Encourage your family member to follow the treatment plan.** Encourage the person to attend treatment sessions regularly. If the medication doesn't seem to help, or the side-effects are uncomfortable, encourage the person to:

- speak to the doctor, nurse or therapist, or another member of the treatment team;
- speak to a pharmacist; or
- get a second opinion.

Go with your relative to an appointment to share your observations. Support your relative's efforts to avoid things that may trigger substance use.

3. **Learn the warning signs of self-harm or suicide.** Warning signs include:

- feeling increasing despair
- winding up affairs
- talking about "When I am gone . . ."

If the person makes any threats, take them very seriously—get help immediately. Call 911 if necessary. Help your family member to see that self-harm or suicidal thinking is a symptom of the illness. Always stress how much you value the person's life.

4. **When your family member is well, plan how to try to avoid crises.** With your family member, work out how to respond to a relapse or crisis. Prepare for how you will deal with:

- a substance use relapse
- an episode of mental health problems
- other potential problems.

5. **Remember your own needs.** Try to:

    - take care of yourself
    - keep up your own support network
    - avoid isolating yourself
    - consider entering therapy for yourself
    - acknowledge the family stresses of coping with concurrent disorders
    - share the responsibility with others, if possible
    - avoid letting the problems take over family life.

6. **Recognize that recovery is slow and gradual.** Know that your family member needs to recover at his or her own pace. You can support recovery from an episode or relapse in these ways:

    - Try not to expect too much, but avoid being overprotective.
    - Try to do things *with* your relative rather than *for* him or her. That way, your relative will slowly regain self-confidence.

7. **See concurrent disorders as an illness, not a character flaw.** Treat your relative normally once he or she has recovered. At the same time, watch for possible signs of relapse. If you see early symptoms, suggest a talk with the care provider.

7 Explaining concurrent disorders to children

Explaining a mental health or substance use problem to children can be awkward and difficult. To protect their children, parents may say nothing. They may try to continue with family routines as if nothing were wrong. This strategy may work in the short term. Over the long term, though, children can feel confused and worried about how their parent's behaviour has changed.

Children are sensitive and intuitive. They quickly notice when someone in the family has changed, particularly a parent. If the family doesn't talk about the problem, children will draw their own, often wrong, conclusions.

Young children, especially those in preschool or early grades, often see the world as revolving around themselves. If something bad happens, they think they caused it. For example, a child may accidentally break something valuable. The next morning, the parent may seem very depressed. The child may then think that breaking the object caused the parent's depression.

A series of pamphlets about talking to children about mental health and substance use problems, entitled *What Kids Want to Know*, is available from the Centre for Addiction and Mental

Health. They list common questions that children have, along with suggestions for how to answer their questions. Online versions are available at http://www.camh.net/Publications/CAMH_Publications/when_parent_pubsindex.html.

How much should I tell the children?

Children need to have things explained. Give them as much information as they can understand.

TODDLERS AND PRESCHOOL CHILDREN

Toddlers and preschool children understand simple, short sentences. They need concrete information and not too much technical language. It is best to explain simply and then try to make the child's life as normal as possible. After explaining the problem, you can make the child feel better if you move on to do something special that the child enjoys.

SCHOOL-AGED CHILDREN

School-aged children can handle more information than younger children. However, they may not understand details about medications and therapies.

TEENAGERS

Teenagers can generally manage most information. Often, they need to talk about their thoughts and feelings. Teenagers worry a lot about what other people, especially their peers, think of themselves and their families. They may ask about genetics. They may also wonder how much they should tell others. They may fear prejudice about mental illness or substance use problems. Sharing information encourages them to talk.

What to tell children

It is helpful to tell the children about three main areas:

1. **The family member has a problem called "concurrent disorders."** The parent or family member behaves this way because he or she is sick. The illness may have symptoms that cause the person's mood or behaviour to change in unpredictable ways.

2. **The child did not cause the problems.** Children need reassurance that they did not make the parent or family member sad, angry or happy. They need to be told that their behaviour did not cause their parent's emotions or behaviour. Children think in concrete terms. If a parent or family member is sad or angry, children can easily feel they did something to cause this, and then feel guilty.

3. **It is not the child's responsibility to make the ill person well.** Children need to know that the adults in the family, and other people, such as doctors, are working to help the person. It is the adults' job to look after the person with the problem.

Children need the well parent and/or other trusted adults to shield them from the effects of the person's symptoms. It is very hard for children to see their parents distressed or in emotional pain. Talking with someone who understands the situation can help sort out the child's confused feelings.

Outside the home

Many children are scared by the changes they see in a family member with concurrent disorders. They miss the time they used to spend with this person. Having activities outside the home helps, because children are exposed to other healthy relationships. As the person recovers, he or she will gradually return to family activities. This can then help mend the relationship between the children and the ill family member.

Parents should talk with their children about what to say to people outside the family. Support from friends is important. However, concurrent disorders can be hard to explain, and some families are concerned that:

- other people will not understand
- other people may act in a way that is prejudiced toward the person with concurrent disorders.

Each family must choose how open it wants to be.

During illness

Children's everyday activities can be noisy. Some people who have concurrent disorders may not be able to tolerate children's noise and behaviour. Family members may need to protect an ill parent from situations that may lead him or her to be irritable and abrupt with the children. At times, children may need to play outside the home. Or the parent may need to rest for part of the day in a quiet area of the house.

During recovery

Once recovered, the parent or other family member can explain his or her behaviour to the children. He or she may need to plan some special times with the children. Such times re-establish the relationship. They reassure the children that the family member is again available and interested in them.

Reference

Reiger, D.A., Farmer, M.E. & Rae, D.S. (1990). Co-morbidity of mental disorders with alcohol and other drug abuse. Results from the Epidemiological Catchment Area (ECA) study. *Journal of the American Medical Association, 264,* 2511–2518.

Resources

GENERAL CONCURRENT DISORDERS

Centre for Addiction and Mental Health
www.camh.net

Health Canada
www.hc-sc.gc.ca/english/search/a-z/a.html

Internet Mental Health
www.mentalhealth.com

Dual Recovery Anonymous
Tel.: 913 991-2703
www.draonline.org

Substance Abuse and Mental Health Services Administration (SAMHSA)
www.samhsa.gov/shin

GENERAL MENTAL HEALTH

CANADA

Canadian Mental Health Association (CMHA)
Tel.: 613 745-7750
www.cmha.ca

Consent and Capacity Board (Ontario)
Tel.: 416 327-4142
Toll-free: 1 866 777-7391
www.ccboard.on.ca

Family Association for Mental Health Everywhere (FAME)
Tel.: 416 207-5032
www.fameforfamilies.com

UNITED STATES

National Alliance on Mental Illness (NAMI)
Information helpline: 1 800 950-6264
www.nami.org

National Institute of Mental Health
www.nimh.nih.gov

National Mental Health Information Center (SAMHSA)
www.mentalhealth.org

INTERNATIONAL

Rethink (U.K.)
www.rethink.org

DEPRESSION

Mood Disorders Association of Ontario
Tel.: 416 486-8046
Toll-free: 1 888 486-8236
www.mooddisorders.on.ca

Depression and Bipolar Support Alliance
Toll-free: 1 800 826-3632
www.dbsalliance.org

ANXIETY

Anxiety Disorders Association of Canada
Tel.: 514 484-0504
Toll-free: 1 888 223-2252
www.anxietycanada.ca

SCHIZOPHRENIA

Schizophrenia Society of Canada
Tel: 204 786-1616
Toll-free: 1 800 263-5545
www.schizophrenia.ca

EATING DISORDERS

National Eating Disorder Information Centre
Tel.: 416 340-4156
Toll-free: 1 866 633 4220
www.nedic.ca

ATTENTION-DEFICIT/HYPERACTIVITY DISORDER

National Resource Center on ADHD (U.S.)
Toll-free: 1 800 233-4050
www.help4adhd.org

GENERAL SUBSTANCE USE

CANADA

Al-Anon/Alateen
www.al-anon.alateen.org

Alcoholics Anonymous
www.aa.org

Narcotics Anonymous
www.na.org

Double Trouble in Recovery
www.doubletroubleinrecovery.org

Canadian Centre on Substance Abuse
www.ccsa.ca

UNITED STATES

National Institute on Drug Abuse (NIDA)
www.nida.nih.gov

CSAT (Center for Substance Abuse Treatment, SAMHSA)
www.samhsa.gov/about/csat.aspx

CSAP (Center for Substance Abuse Prevention SAMHSA)
www.samhsa.gov/prevention

National Clearinghouse on Alcohol and Drug Information (PrevLine)
www.ncadi.samhsa.gov

ONLINE PUBLICATIONS

Best Practices: Concurrent Mental Health and Substance Use Disorders
www.hc-sc.gc.ca/hl-vs/pubs/adp-apd/bp_disorder-mp_concomitants/index_e.html

Report to Congress on the Prevention and Treatment of Co-occurring Substance Abuse Disorders and Mental Disorders (SAMHSA)
www.samhsa.gov/reports/congress2002/index.html

Understanding Psychiatric Medications (CAMH)
www.camh.net/care_treatment/resources_clients_families_friends/psych_meds

Mental Health Medications (U.S. National Institute for Mental Health)
www.nimh.nih.gov/health/publications/mental-health-medications

Expert Consensus Guidelines Series: Guides for Patients and Families
www.psychguides.com

Other guides in this series

Addiction

Anxiety Disorders

Bipolar Disorder

Cognitive-Behavioural Therapy

Couple Therapy

Depressive Illness

First Episode Psychosis

The Forensic Mental Health System in Ontario

Obsessive-Compulsive Disorder

Schizophrenia

Women, Abuse and Trauma Therapy

Women and Psychosis

To order these and other CAMH publications, contact Sales and Distribution:

Tel: 1 800 661-1111
Toronto: 416 595-6059
E-mail: publications@camh.net
Online store: http://store.camh.net